Dummies prediabetes diet

The Complete Guide to manage and reverse Prediabetes with Healthy Recipes

Dr.Stephen Campbell

Table of contents

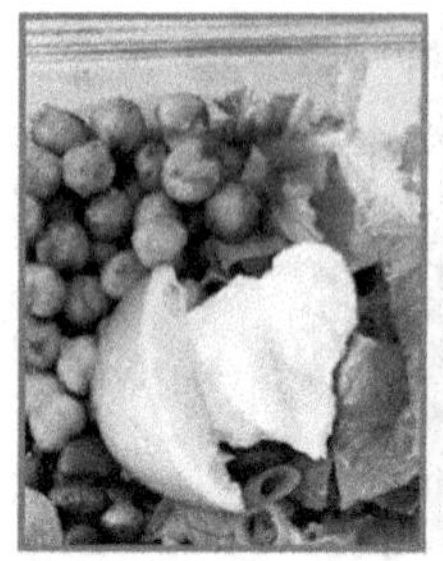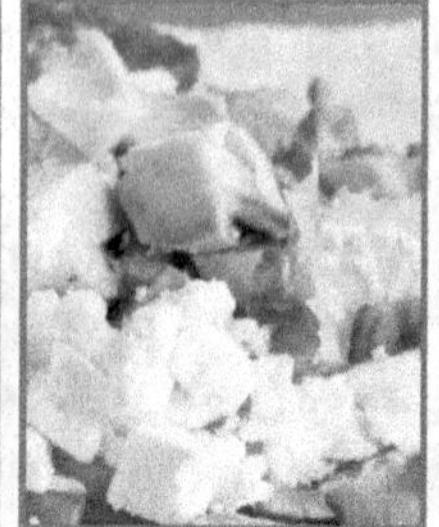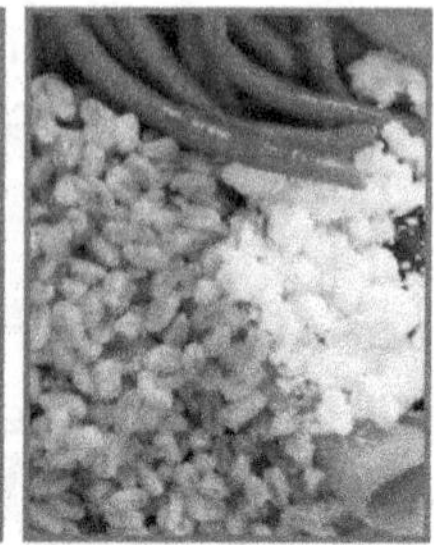

=DUMMIES=
PREDIABETES
DIET

The Complete Guide to manage and reverse
Prediabetes with Healthy Recipes

Dr.Stephen Campbell

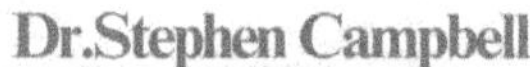

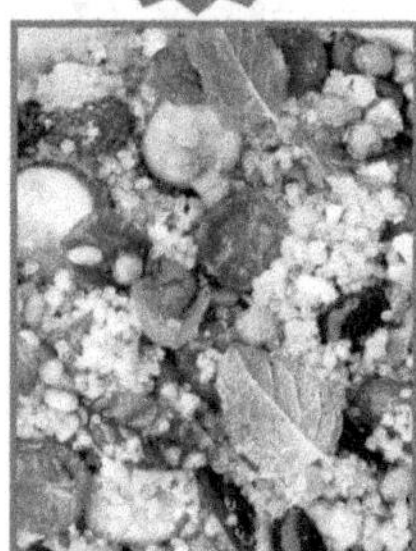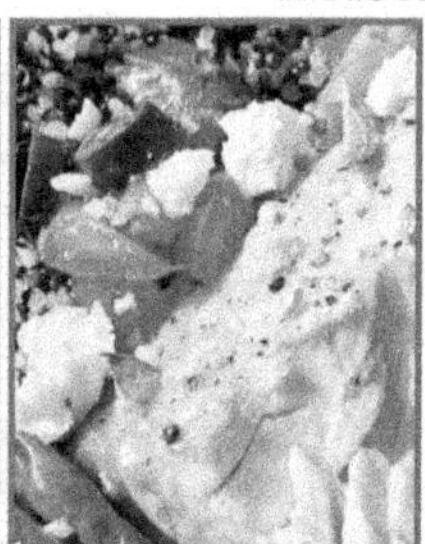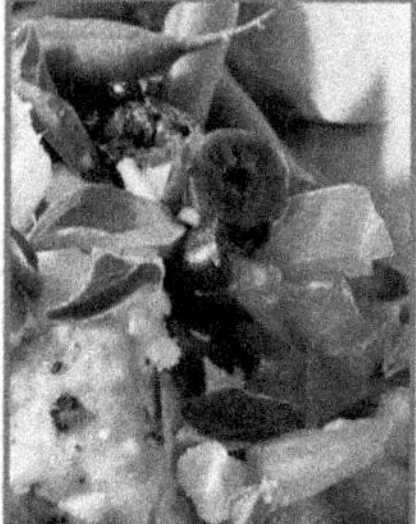

Introduction

In a bustling town, nestled between rolling hills and vibrant meadows, lived a woman named Maya. Maya was known for her boundless energy and radiant smile, but beneath that vivacious exterior, she was facing a silent adversary: prediabetes.

One sunny morning, as Maya strolled through the town market, she overheard a group of villagers whispering about a mysterious healer known as "Elena the Wise." They spoke of her remarkable ability to transform lives through the power of food. Intrigued, Maya decided to seek out this enigmatic healer.

Elena, a kind and gentle soul, welcomed Maya with open arms. Sitting beneath the shade of an ancient oak tree, Elena shared her wisdom. "Maya," she said, "prediabetes is like a shadow that can be tamed with the right tools. And one of the most potent tools we have is the food we eat."

With a sparkle in her eyes, Elena guided Maya through a journey of understanding. She revealed the secrets of nutrient-rich foods that could reverse the course of prediabetes. Leafy greens, vibrant berries, and wholesome grains became Maya's new allies in the battle for her health.

As weeks turned into months, Maya embraced her newfound knowledge and embarked on a culinary adventure. With Elena's guidance, she crafted meals that not only delighted her taste buds but also kept her blood sugar levels in check. Maya's kitchen became a laboratory of transformation, turning fresh ingredients into powerful concoctions of vitality.

Word of Maya's journey spread like wildfire through the town. Friends and neighbors gathered around her table, sharing stories of their own struggles with prediabetes. Together, they discovered the magic of balanced meals and the joy of supporting one another on the path to wellness.

Maya's determination was contagious, and the town began to change. Farmer's markets flourished with colorful produce, and community gardens sprouted like wildflowers. The town's children started a "Healthy Harvest Club," where they learned about the magic of growing their own food.

Through Maya's journey and the wisdom of Elena the Wise, the town not only learned to manage and control prediabetes but also flourished with a newfound vibrancy. The title of "Defeating Prediabetes" was no longer just a book; it had become a mantra of hope and transformation.

And so, Maya's journey became a beacon of light for all those who faced the challenge of prediabetes. With the power of the right diet, they discovered that they held the key to their health and well-being. Just like Maya, they could rewrite their stories, reverse the course of illness, and embrace a life of vitality and joy.

Chapter 1: Understanding Prediabetes

Prediabetes is a wake-up call that should not be ignored. It's a condition characterized by elevated blood sugar levels, indicating an increased risk of developing type 2 diabetes. While it's easy to feel overwhelmed by this diagnosis, knowledge is your most potent weapon against it.

What is Prediabetes?

Prediabetes occurs when the body becomes resistant to the effects of insulin or doesn't produce enough insulin to regulate blood sugar efficiently. This results in higher-than-normal blood sugar levels, but not high enough to be classified as diabetes. However, prediabetes is not a guaranteed path to diabetes. With the right lifestyle changes, it can often be reversed.

Risk Factors for Prediabetes

Several factors contribute to the development of prediabetes, including genetics, weight, inactivity, and age. Individuals with a family history of diabetes, those who are overweight, lead sedentary lifestyles, or are over the age of 45 are at a higher risk. Additionally, certain ethnic groups, such as African Americans, Hispanics, and Native Americans, face an increased predisposition.

Recognizing the Symptoms

Prediabetes often doesn't exhibit noticeable symptoms. However, some individuals may experience unexplained fatigue, increased thirst and hunger, frequent urination, and even darkened skin patches, especially around the neck and armpits. Regular check-ups and blood sugar tests are essential for an accurate diagnosis.

Why Prediabetes Matters

Prediabetes is a critical juncture for intervention. Without lifestyle changes, it can progress to type 2 diabetes, increasing the risk of heart disease, stroke, kidney issues, and nerve damage. The good news is that prediabetes offers an opportunity for positive change. By making healthier choices, you can prevent or delay the onset of diabetes and its associated complications.

This chapter has shed light on what prediabetes is, the risk factors associated with it, and why it matters. Armed with this knowledge, you're ready to explore how dietary changes can play a pivotal role in managing prediabetes and improving your overall well-being.

The Nutritional Magic: Foods that Support Prediabetes Management

Chapter 2: The Nutritional Magic: Foods that Support Prediabetes Management

In the heart of Maya's journey to overcome prediabetes, she learned the profound impact that her diet could have on her health. Guided by Elena the Wise, she uncovered a treasure trove of foods that not only satisfied her taste buds but also played a crucial role in managing her blood sugar levels.

The Power of Whole Grains

Maya bid farewell to refined grains and welcomed whole grains with open arms. Foods like quinoa, brown rice, and whole wheat bread became her staples. Not only did these grains provide sustained energy, but they also prevented rapid spikes in blood sugar. Their fiber content slowed down digestion, keeping

Maya's blood sugar levels stable and her cravings at bay.

Embracing Leafy Greens and Colorful Veggies
Elena introduced Maya to the vibrant world of vegetables, especially leafy greens and colorful veggies. Spinach, kale, broccoli, and bell peppers became her best friends. Packed with vitamins, minerals, and antioxidants, these vegetables supported her body's natural defense against prediabetes. Maya found creative ways to incorporate them into her meals, from hearty salads to flavorful stir-fries.

Berrylicious Delights

Berries were Maya's secret weapon in her battle against prediabetes. Blueberries, strawberries, and raspberries weren't just delicious; they were also low in sugar and high in fiber. Maya enjoyed them in her morning yogurt, as a topping for her oatmeal, or simply as a refreshing snack. The antioxidants in berries helped protect her cells from oxidative stress, a key concern for prediabetes management.

Lean Proteins for Sustained Energy

Protein played a vital role in Maya's journey, as it helped stabilize her blood sugar levels and curb her appetite. Lean sources of protein, such as skinless poultry, fish, tofu, and legumes, became integral parts of her meals. With Elena's guidance, Maya discovered that a well-balanced plate with protein, healthy fats, and fiber-rich carbohydrates was the key to maintaining stable energy levels throughout the day.

Navigating Healthy Fats

Maya bid adieu to trans fats and excessive saturated fats and welcomed healthy fats into her diet. Avocados, nuts, seeds, and olive oil became her sources of nourishing fats. These fats supported her heart health and aided in nutrient absorption. Elena emphasized the importance of portion control, reminding Maya that while fats were beneficial, moderation was key.

Hydration and Herbal Teas

Staying hydrated was another essential aspect of Maya's journey. Water became her constant companion, aiding in digestion and flushing out toxins. Additionally, herbal teas, like cinnamon tea and green tea, offered unique benefits. Cinnamon was known for its potential to improve insulin sensitivity, while green tea's antioxidants boosted overall well-being.

As Maya embraced these dietary changes, she felt a renewed sense of vitality. Her energy levels soared, her moods stabilized, and most importantly, her blood sugar levels started to show improvement. With each meal, Maya was making a conscious choice to nourish her body and support her goal of reversing prediabetes

Chapter 3: Crafting Your Prediabetes Diet Plan

As Maya delved deeper into her journey of managing prediabetes through diet, she realized that a well-structured meal plan was essential for success. With Elena's guidance, she embarked on the art of meal crafting, ensuring that each bite she took was a step towards better health.

The Balanced Plate Approach

Elena introduced Maya to the concept of the balanced plate. Each meal was a canvas where Maya could paint a masterpiece of nutrients. Half of her plate was dedicated to colorful vegetables, a quarter to lean proteins, and the remaining quarter to whole grains or starchy vegetables. This approach ensured a harmonious balance of nutrients that kept her blood sugar levels steady.

Portion Control and Mindful Eating

Maya learned that portion control was just as important as the foods she chose. Through mindful eating, she began to listen to her body's cues of hunger and fullness. She savored each bite, chewed slowly, and put her fork down between bites. This allowed her to enjoy her meals more fully and prevented overeating.

The Importance of Regular Meals

Gone were the days of skipping meals or going long periods without eating. Maya understood that consistent meal timing was crucial for managing blood sugar levels. She aimed to have three balanced meals and two healthy snacks throughout the day. This approach prevented extreme spikes and crashes in her blood sugar, providing a steady source of energy.

Prepping for Success

Maya discovered the beauty of meal prepping, a practice that saved time and ensured that she always had healthy options at her fingertips. She spent a portion of her weekend washing, chopping, and cooking ingredients for the week ahead. With prepped veggies, cooked grains, and marinated proteins, creating a balanced meal was a breeze, even on the busiest days.

Mindful Indulgences

Elena reminded Maya that an occasional treat was part of a sustainable prediabetes diet. Maya learned to indulge mindfully, savoring each bite and appreciating the flavors. She found healthier alternatives for her favorite treats, like dark chocolate or homemade fruit sorbet. By practicing moderation and balance,

Maya could enjoy her favorite indulgences without derailing her progress.

Keeping a Food Diary

To keep track of her meals and understand how they affected her blood sugar levels, Maya started a food diary. This simple practice allowed her to identify patterns and make informed choices. If certain foods cause undesirable spikes, she knows to adjust her portions or opt for alternatives.

With her prediabetes diet plan in place, Maya felt empowered. Each meal was a chance to nourish her body and take control of her health. As she embraced the balanced plate, portion control, and mindful eating, she witnessed her blood sugar levels becoming more stable. The journey wasn't always easy, but Maya knew that every choice she made was a step closer to her goal of defeating prediabetes.

Chapter 4: Your Prediabetes-Friendly Grocery Shopping Guide

As Maya's journey to manage prediabetes through diet continued, she realized that a well-curated grocery list was the foundation of her success. With Elena's guidance, Maya developed a professional diet plan that included a variety of prediabetes-friendly foods. Here's a sample of what Maya's weekly grocery list and diet plan looked like:

Weekly Grocery List:

Proteins:

- Skinless chicken breasts
- Turkey breast
- Salmon fillets
- Tofu
- Lentils

Vegetables:

- Spinach
- Kale
- Broccoli
- Bell peppers
- Zucchini
- Tomatoes

Fruits:

- Blueberries
- Strawberries
- Apples
- Oranges
- Avocado

Grains:

- Quinoa
- Brown rice
- Whole wheat bread
- Rolled oats

Dairy and Alternatives:

- Greek yogurt (unsweetened)
- Almond milk (unsweetened)

Nuts and Seeds:

- Almonds
- Walnuts
- Chia seeds

- **Pantry Staples:**
- Olive oil
- Balsamic vinegar
- Herbs and spices (cinnamon, turmeric, cumin, etc.)
- Whole grain pasta

Snacks:

- Carrot sticks
- Hummus
- Rice cakes

Sample Diet Plan:

Breakfast:
- Greek yogurt with a handful of blueberries and a sprinkle of chia seeds
- Avocado slices on whole grain toast with a poached egg

Morning Snack:
- Apple slices and a few of almonds

Lunch:
- Grilled chicken salad with a mix of spinach, kale, bell peppers, and tomatoes
- Quinoa as a base, dressed with olive oil and balsamic vinegar

Afternoon Snack:
- Carrot sticks with hummus

Dinner:

- Baked salmon fillet with a side of roasted broccoli and brown rice
- A side salad with mixed greens, strawberries, and a light vinaigrette

Evening Snack:
- Orange slices

Maya's diet plan focused on nutrient-dense foods that supported stable blood sugar levels. Lean proteins provided sustained energy, while colorful vegetables and fruits supplied essential vitamins and antioxidants. Whole grains and fiber-rich foods prevented rapid spikes in blood sugar, promoting overall health.

Elena advised Maya to stay hydrated by drinking plenty of water throughout the day. Additionally, she encouraged Maya to experiment with herbs and spices to add flavor to her dishes without relying on excessive salt or sugar.

Maya's journey was a testament to the power of a well-thought-out diet plan. With each meal, she was taking steps towards better health and defeating prediabetes. In the next chapter, we'll explore the art of meal prepping, as Maya learns to prepare her ingredients in advance and create balanced meals even on the busiest of days. Get ready to master the art of nourishment and efficiency!

Chapter 5: Mastering the Art of Meal Prepping for Prediabetes Management

As Maya continued on her path to managing prediabetes through diet, she recognized the importance of efficiency in maintaining her newfound healthy eating habits. With Elena's guidance, she delved into the world of meal prepping – a skill that not only saved time but also ensured that her meals aligned with her health goals.

The Benefits of Meal Prepping:

Meal prepping offered Maya a range of benefits:

Time-Saving: With ingredients prepped in advance, Maya spent less time chopping and cooking during the week.

Consistent Portions: Portion control was easier, as Maya could measure out her servings ahead of time.

Healthy Choices: Having prediabetes-friendly meals ready prevented impulsive, less nutritious choices.

Less Stress: Busy days were easier to navigate, knowing that a balanced meal was just a reheat away.

Getting Started:

Maya set aside time on Sundays for her meal prepping sessions. She invested in a variety of meal prep containers in different sizes, making it easy to portion out her ingredients.

Step-by-Step Meal Prepping:

1. Plan Your Meals:

Maya reviewed her diet plan and selected recipes for the week. She ensured each meal had a balance of proteins, vegetables, and whole grains.

2. Grocery Shopping:

Armed with her grocery list, Maya purchased all the ingredients she needed for her chosen recipes.

3. Wash and Chop Veggies:

Back home, Maya washed, peeled, and chopped her vegetables. She separated them into containers based on their use – some for salads, some for stir-fries, and others for snacks.

4. Cook Proteins and Grains:

Maya cooked her proteins (chicken, turkey, tofu) and grains (quinoa, brown rice) in bulk. She seasoned them lightly to allow for versatility in flavors.

5. Assemble Meals:

Using her meal prep containers, Maya assembled her meals. Each container contained a protein source, vegetables, and a serving of grains.

6. Snack Packs:

Maya created snack packs by portioning out nuts, seeds, and cut fruits. These were perfect for her mid-morning and afternoon snacks.

7. Label and Store:

Maya labeled her containers with the meal type and date. She stored them in the fridge, making sure that items she planned to use later in the week were placed towards the back.

Enjoying the Fruits of Meal Prepping:
Throughout the week, Maya relished the convenience of her prepped meals. Mornings were stress-free with breakfast options at the ready, and lunches were a breeze to pack for work. Evenings were relaxed, as dinner came together in a matter of minutes.

With meal prepping as her ally, Maya seamlessly integrated healthy eating into her lifestyle. She marveled at how a few hours of planning and preparation transformed her relationship with food. In the next chapter, Maya will explore the realm of breakfast options, discovering delicious and nourishing ways to start her day on the right foot. Get ready to wake up to a prediabetes-friendly morning routine!

Breakfasts that Fuel Your Day:

Chapter 6: Breakfasts that Fuel Your Day: Prediabetes-Friendly Morning Options

Maya's journey to manage prediabetes through diet brought her to a crucial realization — breakfast was not just a meal; it was the foundation of her day. With Elena's guidance, she explored a variety of prediabetes-friendly breakfast options, ensuring that her mornings began on the right note.

The Importance of a Balanced Breakfast:

Elena emphasized that a balanced breakfast was essential for stable blood sugar levels throughout the day. Maya's breakfasts were designed to include a mix of lean proteins, fiber-rich carbohydrates, and healthy fats.

Prediabetes-Friendly Breakfast Ideas:

1. Greek Yogurt Parfait:

A bowl of Greek yogurt topped with fresh berries, a drizzle of honey, and a sprinkle of chopped nuts. This parfait was a delightful blend of flavors and textures, offering protein, antioxidants, and healthy fats.

2. Veggie Omelette:

A fluffy omelette filled with sautéed vegetables like spinach, bell peppers, and tomatoes. Maya often paired it with a slice of whole grain toast for a complete meal.

3. Overnight Oats:

A jar filled with rolled oats, almond milk, chia seeds, and a touch of cinnamon. Maya left it in the fridge overnight, and in the morning, she added sliced bananas and a dollop of almond butter for a satisfying start to her day.

4. Smoothie Bowl:

A thick and vibrant smoothie bowl made with spinach, frozen berries, a scoop of protein powder, and almond milk. Maya topped it with granola, sliced almonds, and a sprinkle of coconut flakes.

5. Avocado Toast with Egg:

Mashed avocado spread on whole grain toast, topped with a poached egg and a pinch of red pepper flakes. The healthy fats in avocado and the protein in the egg provided lasting energy.

6. Chia Seed Pudding:

A creamy chia seed pudding made by mixing chia seeds with almond milk and letting it sit in the fridge overnight. In the morning, Maya added sliced fruits and a drizzle of honey.

Morning Rituals for Success:

Maya embraced her morning routine as a time of nourishment and reflection. She started her day with a glass of water to rehydrate her body. After enjoying her prediabetes-friendly breakfast, she took a few moments to practice deep breathing or light stretching, setting a positive tone for the day ahead.

Through her breakfast choices, Maya found a renewed sense of energy and focus. Her mornings became a time of mindful nourishment, and her blood sugar levels remained stable throughout the day. In the next chapter, Maya will explore the world of healthy lunch options, discovering ways to stay satisfied and energized as she navigates her busy afternoons. Get ready to uncover the art of prediabetes-friendly lunches!

Chapter 7: Nourishing Your Midday: Healthy Lunches for Stable Blood Sugar

Maya's journey to manage prediabetes through diet continued to evolve, and her focus shifted to mastering the art of crafting prediabetes-friendly lunches. With Elena's guidance, Maya explored a variety of lunch options that kept her energy levels steady and her blood sugar in check.

The Lunchtime Balancing Act:

Elena reminded Maya that a balanced lunch was essential for preventing mid-afternoon crashes and maintaining her overall well-being. Maya's lunches were designed to provide sustained energy through a combination of lean proteins, fiber-rich carbohydrates, and a rainbow of vegetables.

Prediabetes-Friendly Lunch Ideas:

1. Grilled Chicken Salad:

A colorful salad made with grilled chicken breast, mixed greens, cherry tomatoes, cucumber slices, and a light vinaigrette dressing. Maya often added a sprinkle of nuts or seeds for added crunch.

2. Quinoa and Veggie Bowl:

A bowl filled with cooked quinoa, sautéed vegetables, and a serving of lean protein like tofu or beans. Maya drizzled olive oil and lemon juice for extra flavor.

3. Whole Grain Wrap:

A whole wheat wrap filled with lean turkey slices, hummus, and a variety of colorful veggies. Maya rolled it up and enjoyed it with a side of carrot sticks.

4. Lentil Soup and Side Salad:

A hearty bowl of lentil soup served with a side salad of mixed greens, bell peppers, and a sprinkle of feta cheese. Maya paired it with a slice of whole grain bread.

5. Stir-Fried Tofu and Veggies:

Tofu and an array of vegetables stir-fried in a light sesame oil and soy sauce. Maya served it over a bed of brown rice for a satisfying meal.

6. Mediterranean Plate:

A plate featuring hummus, whole wheat pita bread, olives, cherry tomatoes, and cucumber slices. Maya added a few grilled shrimp for protein.

Lunchtime Rituals for Success:

Maya transformed her lunch break into a time of mindful nourishment. She found a peaceful spot to enjoy her meal without distractions. After eating, she took a short stroll to help with digestion and boost her energy for the rest of the day.

Maya's prediabetes-friendly lunches not only kept her blood sugar stable but also fueled her productivity and focus. As she continued to experiment with different lunch options, Maya marveled at how small changes could lead to significant improvements in her well-being. In the next chapter, Maya will explore the realm of nutritious snacks, discovering ways to keep her energy levels up between meals. Get ready to uncover the art of snacking for prediabetes management!

Chapter 8: Smart Snacking Strategies: Nourishing Prediabetes-Friendly Snack Choices

Maya's journey to manage prediabetes through diet reached a pivotal point as she delved into the world of smart snacking. With Elena's guidance, Maya learned that well-chosen snacks could help maintain stable blood sugar levels and provide a boost of energy between meals.

The Power of Mindful Snacking:

Elena stressed the importance of mindful snacking – choosing nutrient-dense options that aligned with Maya's health goals. Maya's snacks were designed to include a combination of protein, fiber, and healthy fats, helping her stay satisfied and preventing blood sugar spikes.

Prediabetes-Friendly Snack Ideas:

1. Apple Slices with Nut Butter:

Crisp apple slices paired with a dollop of almond or peanut butter. The combination of fiber from the apple and healthy fats from the nut butter provided sustained energy.

2. Greek Yogurt and Berries:

a little dish of Greek yogurt with some fresh berries on top. Maya sometimes added a sprinkle of granola for added crunch.

3. Veggie Sticks with Hummus:

Carrot, celery, and cucumber sticks served with a portion of hummus. The fiber from the veggies and the protein from the hummus kept Maya feeling full and satisfied.

4. Trail Mix with Nuts and Seeds:

A small handful of mixed nuts and seeds, such as almonds, walnuts, and pumpkin seeds. This snack provided healthy fats and a satisfying crunch.

5. Rice Cakes with Avocado:

Lightly salted rice cakes topped with mashed avocado and a sprinkle of black pepper. The healthy fats in avocado helped stabilize blood sugar levels.

6. Cottage Cheese with Pineapple:

Low-fat cottage cheese paired with a few pineapple chunks. This snack offered a combination of protein and natural sweetness.

Snacking with Intention:

Maya learned to snack with intention, paying attention to her body's signals of hunger and fullness. She kept her snacks portion-controlled and avoided mindless munching while watching TV or working on her computer.

By incorporating prediabetes-friendly snacks into her routine, Maya maintained her energy levels throughout the day. She felt empowered by her ability to make nourishing choices even during moments of hunger. In the next chapter, Maya will explore the realm of wholesome dinners, discovering ways to end her day with a satisfying and balanced meal. Get ready to uncover the art of prediabetes-friendly dinners!

Chapter 9: Wholesome Dinners for Prediabetes Management: Savoring Balanced Evening Meals

Maya's journey to manage prediabetes through diet entered a crucial phase as she turned her attention to crafting wholesome dinners. With Elena's guidance, Maya discovered that ending her day with a balanced and nourishing meal was essential for maintaining stable blood sugar levels and promoting overall well-being.

The Importance of Dinners in Prediabetes Management:

Elena emphasized that dinners played a significant role in Maya's prediabetes journey. A well-structured dinner could prevent overeating later in the evening and ensure that Maya woke up with stable blood sugar levels.

Prediabetes-Friendly Dinner Ideas:

1. Grilled Vegetable and Chicken Stir-Fry:

A colorful stir-fry made with grilled chicken, an array of colorful vegetables, and a light soy-ginger sauce. Maya served it over a small portion of brown rice or quinoa.

2. Baked Salmon with Roasted Vegetables:

A flaky baked salmon filet paired with roasted broccoli, carrots, and cauliflower. Maya drizzled olive oil and added her favorite herbs and spices for flavor.

3. Lentil and Spinach Curry:

A hearty lentil and spinach curry served with a side of whole grain naan or brown rice. The combination of protein and fiber kept Maya satisfied.

4. Turkey and Veggie Stuffed Bell Peppers:

Bell peppers stuffed with a mixture of lean ground turkey, quinoa, diced tomatoes, and spices. Maya baked them until tender and enjoyed a colorful and flavorful meal.

5. Tofu and Broccoli Quinoa Bowl:

Pan-seared tofu served with steamed broccoli and quinoa. Maya drizzled a homemade tahini dressing over the bowl for added creaminess.

6. Eggplant and Chickpea Ratatouille:

A comforting ratatouille made with eggplant, zucchini, bell peppers, and chickpeas. Maya enjoyed it as a warm and satisfying dinner.

Creating Dinner Rituals:

Maya transformed dinner into a mindful and peaceful ritual. She set the table with care, creating an ambiance that encouraged her to savor each bite. Maya also made it a habit to eat dinner at a consistent time, allowing her body to regulate its blood sugar levels more effectively.

Through her pre diabetes-friendly dinners, Maya discovered that nourishing choices could be both satisfying and delicious. With each meal, she nurtured her body and supported her goal of managing prediabetes. In the next chapter, Maya will explore strategies for navigating social events and eating out while staying true to her health journey. Get ready to uncover the art of mindful choices in social settings!

Chapter 10: Navigating Social Events and Eating Out: Making Mindful Choices

Maya's journey to manage prediabetes through diet reached a point where she needed to navigate social events and dining out while staying true to her health goals. With Elena's guidance, Maya learned how to make mindful choices in various settings without compromising her progress.

The Challenge of Social Settings:

Elena acknowledged that social events and dining out could present challenges, but they also offered opportunities for Maya to practice her newfound knowledge about prediabetes-friendly eating.

Mindful Choices at Social Events:

1. Prioritize Portions: Maya chose smaller portions of high-carb dishes and focused on lean proteins and vegetables.

2. Opt for Whole Grains: When available, Maya chose whole grain options like brown rice or whole wheat pasta.

3. Fill Up on Veggies: Maya loaded her plate with colorful vegetables to ensure a balanced meal.

4. Limit Sugary Drinks: Maya opted for water, sparkling water, or unsweetened iced tea instead of sugary beverages.

Dining Out with Intent:
1. Check the Menu Ahead: Maya reviewed menus online before going out to make informed choices.

2. Customization: Maya wasn't afraid to ask for modifications, like swapping fries for a side salad.

3. Choose Grilled or Baked: Maya opted for grilled, baked, or steamed dishes instead of fried options.

4. Dressing on the Side: Maya requested dressings and sauces on the side to control portions.

5. Share Desserts: If dessert was on the menu, Maya shared it with friends to enjoy a few bites without overindulging.

Enjoying Every Bite:
Elena reminded Maya that the goal was not perfection but balance. Maya learned to savor each bite, enjoying the flavors and the company of those around her. If she occasionally indulged, she did so mindfully and without guilt.

Maya's ability to make mindful choices in social settings and while dining out showcased her commitment to her health journey. She realized that she had the power to enjoy these moments without compromising her prediabetes management goals. In the next chapter, Maya will delve into the importance of incorporating physical activity into her routine, discovering how movement could further support her well-being. Get ready to explore the art of an active lifestyle!

Chapter 11: Embracing an Active Lifestyle: Movement for Prediabetes Wellness

Maya's journey to manage prediabetes through diet expanded to incorporate the importance of an active lifestyle. With Elena's guidance, Maya discovered the transformative effects of physical activity and how it could further enhance her well-being.

The Role of Physical Activity:

Elena explained that regular physical activity played a crucial role in managing prediabetes. It helped improve insulin sensitivity, lower blood sugar levels, and support overall heart health.

Designing an Active Routine:

1. Choose Activities You Enjoy: Maya explored various activities, from walking and swimming

to dancing and yoga, to find what resonated with her.

2. Set Realistic Goals: Maya started with achievable goals, gradually increasing the intensity and duration of her workouts.

3. Mix Cardio and Strength Training: Maya balanced cardiovascular exercises like brisk walking with strength training routines.

4. Prioritize Consistency: Maya aimed for regularity, setting aside specific times for physical activity each day.

Incorporating Movement into Daily Life:

1. Walk More: Maya incorporated more walking into her routine by parking farther away, taking the stairs, or going for short walks during breaks.

2. Active Commuting: When possible, Maya walked or biked for short commutes, adding more movement to her day.

3. Desk Stretches: Maya performed simple stretches at her desk to relieve tension and maintain flexibility.

4. Family Activities: Maya involved her family in activities like hiking, playing sports, or having dance parties at home.

Mind and Body Connection:

Maya learned that physical activity wasn't just about the body — it also benefited her mental and emotional well-being. Movement became a way for her to release stress, boost her mood, and feel more energized.

Tracking Progress:

Maya tracked her progress, noting improvements in her endurance, strength, and flexibility. This sense of achievement motivated her to continue her active lifestyle.

A Journey of Movement:

As Maya embraced an active lifestyle, she felt a renewed sense of vitality and empowerment. Each step, each stretch, and each moment of movement was a testament to her commitment to managing prediabetes and living a healthier life. In the next chapter, Maya will explore the importance of restorative sleep and its impact on her overall well-being. Get ready to uncover the art of a good night's sleep!

Chapter 12: The Power of Restful Sleep: Prioritizing Sleep for Prediabetes Wellness

Maya's journey to manage prediabetes through diet and an active lifestyle expanded to encompass the importance of restful sleep. With Elena's guidance, Maya delved into the world of sleep and discovered how it could profoundly impact her overall well-being.

Understanding the Sleep Connection:

Elena explained that sleep played a crucial role in managing prediabetes. Quality sleep supported hormone regulation, improved insulin sensitivity, and contributed to overall metabolic health.

Creating a Sleep-Friendly Environment:

1. Set a Consistent Schedule: Maya aimed to go to bed and wake up at the same times each day to regulate her body's internal clock.

2. Create a Relaxing Bedtime Routine: Maya practiced calming activities before bed, such as reading, gentle stretching, or deep breathing.

3. Comfortable Sleep Environment: Maya ensured her sleep environment was conducive to rest – a comfortable mattress, soft bedding, and a cool room.

4. Limit Screen Time: Maya avoided screens at least an hour before bed, as the blue light could disrupt her sleep cycle.

Nurturing a Healthy Sleep Routine:

1. Balanced Meals: Maya avoided heavy meals close to bedtime, opting for a light snack if needed.

2. Hydration: Maya stayed hydrated throughout the day but limited liquids in the evening to prevent nighttime awakenings.

3. Physical Activity: Maya engaged in regular physical activity, which contributed to better sleep quality.

4. Stress Management: Maya practiced relaxation techniques, such as meditation or gentle yoga, to ease her mind before bed.

Unveiling the Benefits of Restorative Sleep:

As Maya prioritized restful sleep, she noticed improvements in her energy levels, mood, and overall well-being. Her blood sugar levels became more stable, and she felt more equipped to tackle the challenges of her prediabetes journey.

Maya's commitment to nurturing her sleep taught her that self-care extended beyond diet and exercise. It encompassed every aspect of her life, including the vital act of getting enough rest. In the next chapter, Maya will explore the art of managing stress and maintaining a positive mindset in her journey towards prediabetes wellness. Get ready to uncover the strategies for cultivating resilience and emotional balance!

Chapter 13: Cultivating Resilience: Managing Stress and Embracing Positivity

Maya's journey to manage prediabetes through diet, exercise, sleep, and mindful choices led her to the realization that emotional well-being played a vital role in her overall health. With Elena's guidance, Maya explored strategies to manage stress, cultivate resilience, and embrace positivity.

The Mind-Body Connection:

Elena explained that stress could impact blood sugar levels and overall health. Maya learned that managing stress was an essential component of her prediabetes journey.

Stress-Reducing Techniques:

1. Mindfulness Meditation: Maya practiced mindfulness meditation to stay present and reduce anxiety.

2. Deep Breathing: Maya used deep breathing exercises to calm her mind during moments of stress.

3. Journaling: Maya kept a journal to express her thoughts and emotions, gaining insight and clarity.

4. Nature Walks: Maya enjoyed spending time in nature, taking leisurely walks to clear her mind.

Cultivating Positivity:

1. Gratitude Practice: Maya started each day by listing things she was grateful for, fostering a positive outlook.

2. Positive Affirmations: Maya used positive affirmations to counter negative self-talk and boost her confidence.

3. Surrounding Yourself: Maya surrounded herself with supportive and positive individuals who uplifted her.

Creating Emotional Resilience:

Maya understood that setbacks were part of her journey, but she learned to view them as opportunities for growth. She embraced challenges with a mindset of curiosity and a determination to learn from every experience.

Mind and Body Harmony:

Maya's efforts to manage stress and cultivate positivity enhanced her overall well-being. She noticed that as her emotional health improved, her physical health followed suit. The mind-body connection was a powerful force in her journey towards prediabetes wellness.

In the next chapter, Maya will explore the concept of long-term sustainability, discovering how she can continue to thrive and maintain her prediabetes-friendly lifestyle for years to come. Get ready to uncover the art of lasting wellness!

Chapter 14: Sustaining Your Wellness Journey: Long-Term Strategies for Prediabetes Management

Maya's journey to manage prediabetes through diet, exercise, sleep, and emotional well-being had brought her a long way. With Elena's guidance, Maya delved into the world of long-term sustainability, discovering strategies that would help her maintain her prediabetes-friendly lifestyle for years to come.

The Road to Lasting Wellness:

Elena explained that the key to long-term success was creating habits that became an integral part of Maya's life, rather than temporary changes.

Lifestyle Over Diets:

Maya shifted her perspective from "dieting" to adopting a sustainable lifestyle. She focused on making gradual, consistent changes that she could maintain in the long run.

Staying Curious and Open:

Maya continued to explore new foods, recipes, and activities. She embraced a sense of curiosity, knowing that her wellness journey was an ongoing adventure.

Goal Setting and Tracking:

Maya set realistic goals for herself and tracked her progress. Celebrating even the smallest victories kept her motivated and encouraged.

Adapting to Change:

Maya learned that life could be unpredictable, and her wellness journey needed to be flexible. She developed strategies to adapt her habits during busy times or unexpected events.

Social Support:

Maya found a community of like-minded individuals who supported her wellness goals. Whether online or in person, connecting with others provided a sense of accountability and encouragement.

Self-Compassion:
Maya practiced self-compassion, recognizing that setbacks were normal and not a reason to give up. She treated herself with kindness and patience.

Reflecting and Celebrating:
Maya took moments to reflect on how far she had come and celebrated her achievements. Recognizing her growth reinforced her commitment to her well-being.

Embracing the Journey:
Maya realized that her prediabetes-friendly lifestyle was not just a means to an end but a continuous journey of self-care and growth.

Each day was an opportunity to make choices that aligned with her health and happiness.

As Maya embraced the art of lasting wellness, she felt empowered to continue thriving on her prediabetes journey. In the final chapter, Maya will reflect on her transformation, celebrating her achievements and looking towards a future of vibrant health and well-being. Get ready to witness the culmination of Maya's incredible journey!

Chapter 15: Celebrating Transformation: A Future of Vibrant Health and Well-Being

Maya's transformative journey to manage prediabetes through diet, exercise, sleep, emotional well-being, and sustainable choices had led her to a place of vibrant health and well-being. With Elena's guidance, Maya reflected on her incredible transformation and looked ahead to a future filled with possibilities.

A Journey of Growth:

Maya marveled at how far she had come since the beginning of her prediabetes journey. She recognized that her dedication and commitment had led to remarkable changes in her health and overall quality of life.

Reflecting on Achievements:

Maya took time to celebrate her achievements – from adopting a balanced diet to embracing physical activity, improving her sleep, managing stress, and cultivating a positive mindset.

Empowerment Through Knowledge:
Maya's journey was characterized by empowerment through knowledge. The more she learned about prediabetes and wellness, the more in control she felt of her health and future.

A Vision of the Future:
Looking ahead, Maya felt a sense of excitement about the possibilities that lay before her. She envisioned a life filled with continued growth, vibrant health, and a deep appreciation for every moment.

Inspiring Others:
Maya's transformation inspired those around her. Her friends, family, and even strangers

were motivated by her dedication and success, making positive changes in their own lives.

A Life Well-Lived:

Maya's journey was not just about managing prediabetes; it was about living a life that aligned with her values and well-being. She realized that every choice she made was an opportunity to nurture her body, mind, and spirit.

A Note to Fellow Journeyers:

Maya left a heartfelt note for those who were embarking on their own prediabetes journeys. She shared words of encouragement, reminding them that the path to wellness was not always linear, but every step forward mattered.

As Maya closed this chapter of her journey, she looked towards the horizon with a heart full of gratitude and anticipation. The art of managing prediabetes had transformed her life in profound ways, reminding her that she possessed the power to create her own future of vibrant health and well-being.

And so, with a deep sense of accomplishment and excitement, Maya stepped forward into her future – a future shaped by her journey, her choices, and her unwavering commitment to living a life of vitality and purpose.

The End

Bonus : "Delicious Pre Diabetes-Friendly Recipes: Nourishing Your Body with Flavor"

Prediabetes-Friendly Recipes:

Breakfast:

Greek Yogurt Parfait:

- Greek yogurt, mixed berries, honey, chopped nuts
- Nutritional Info: Calories: 250, Carbs: 30g, Protein: 15g, Fat: 8g, Fiber: 5g

Spinach and Mushroom Omelette:

- Eggs, spinach, mushrooms, onions, feta cheese
- Nutritional Info: Calories: 280, Carbs: 8g, Protein: 18g, Fat: 20g, Fiber: 2g

Overnight Chia Pudding:

- Chia seeds, almond milk, berries, almonds
- Nutritional Info: Calories: 220, Carbs: 20g, Protein: 8g, Fat: 14g, Fiber: 12g

Whole Grain Pancakes:

- Whole wheat flour, Greek yogurt, berries, maple syrup
- Nutritional Info: Calories: 290, Carbs: 40g, Protein: 15g, Fat: 8g, Fiber: 6g

Avocado Toast with Poached Egg:

- Whole grain bread, avocado, poached egg, red pepper flakes
- Nutritional Info: Calories: 320, Carbs: 25g, Protein: 15g, Fat: 20g, Fiber: 10g

Lunch:

Grilled Chicken Salad:

- Grilled chicken, mixed greens, veggies, vinaigrette

- Nutritional Info: Calories: 350, Carbs: 20g, Protein: 30g, Fat: 15g, Fiber: 5g

Quinoa and Veggie Bowl:
- Quinoa, mixed veggies, tofu, olive oil, lemon
- Nutritional Info: Calories: 380, Carbs: 45g, Protein: 18g, Fat: 15g, Fiber: 8g

Lentil Soup with Side Salad:
- Lentil soup, mixed greens, veggies, light dressing
- Nutritional Info: Calories: 300, Carbs: 40g, Protein: 15g, Fat: 8g, Fiber: 10g

Turkey and Hummus Wrap:
- Whole wheat wrap, lean turkey, hummus, veggies
- Nutritional Info: Calories: 320, Carbs: 30g, Protein: 25g, Fat: 12g, Fiber: 6g

Quinoa and Black Bean Salad:

- Quinoa, black beans, corn, bell peppers, lime dressing
- Nutritional Info: Calories: 280, Carbs: 45g, Protein: 10g, Fat: 6g, Fiber: 8g

Snacks:
- Apple Slices with Nut Butter:
- Apple slices, almond butter
- Nutritional Info: Calories: 180, Carbs: 20g, Protein: 4g, Fat: 10g, Fiber: 5g

Greek Yogurt and Berries:
- Greek yogurt, mixed berries
- Nutritional Info: Calories: 150, Carbs: 15g, Protein: 10g, Fat: 5g, Fiber: 3g

Carrot Sticks with Hummus:
- Carrot sticks, hummus
- Nutritional Info: Calories: 120, Carbs: 15g, Protein: 4g, Fat: 6g, Fiber: 4g

Trail Mix:
- Mixed nuts, seeds, dried fruit

- Nutritional Info: Calories: 200, Carbs: 15g, Protein: 6g, Fat: 14g, Fiber: 4g

Cottage Cheese with Pineapple:
- Low-fat cottage cheese, pineapple
- Nutritional Info: Calories: 150, Carbs: 20g, Protein: 12g, Fat: 2g, Fiber: 2g

Dinner:

Grilled Vegetable and Chicken Stir-Fry:
- Grilled chicken, assorted veggies, soy-ginger sauce
- Nutritional Info: Calories: 350, Carbs: 25g, Protein: 30g, Fat: 12g, Fiber: 8g

Baked Salmon with Roasted Vegetables:
- Baked salmon, roasted veggies, olive oil, herbs
- Nutritional Info: Calories: 380, Carbs: 20g, Protein: 30g, Fat: 18g, Fiber: 8g

Lentil and Spinach Curry:
- Lentils, spinach, tomatoes, curry spices

- Nutritional Info: Calories: 300, Carbs: 40g, Protein: 15g, Fat: 8g, Fiber: 12g

Tofu and Broccoli Quinoa Bowl:
- Pan-seared tofu, steamed broccoli, quinoa, tahini dressing
- Nutritional Info: Calories: 380, Carbs: 40g, Protein: 20g, Fat: 15g, Fiber: 8g

- Eggplant and Chickpea Ratatouille:
- Eggplant, chickpeas, assorted veggies, Mediterranean spices
- Nutritional Info: Calories: 320, Carbs: 45g, Protein: 12g, Fat: 10g, Fiber: 10g

7-Day Pre Diabetes-Friendly Meal Plan:

Day 1:
Breakfast: Greek Yogurt Parfait
Lunch: Grilled Chicken Salad

Snack: Carrot Sticks with Hummus

Dinner: Lentil and Spinach Curry

Day 2:

Breakfast: Spinach and Mushroom Omelette

Lunch: Quinoa and Black Bean Salad

Snack: Cottage Cheese with Pineapple

Dinner: Baked Salmon with Roasted Vegetables

Day 3:

Breakfast: Overnight Chia Pudding

Lunch: Turkey and Hummus Wrap

Snack: Apple Slices with Nut Butter

Dinner: Eggplant and Chickpea Ratatouille

Day 4:

Breakfast: Avocado Toast with Poached Egg

Lunch: Quinoa and Veggie Bowl

Snack: Greek Yogurt and Berries

Dinner: Grilled Vegetable and Chicken Stir-Fry

Day 5:

Breakfast: Whole Grain Pancakes

Lunch: Lentil Soup with Side Salad

Snack: Trail Mix

Dinner: Tofu and Broccoli Quinoa Bowl

Day 6:

Breakfast: Greek Yogurt Parfait

Lunch: Grilled Chicken Salad

Snack: Carrot Sticks with Hummus

Dinner: Lentil and Spinach Curry

Day 7:

Breakfast: Spinach and Mushroom Omelette

Lunch: Quinoa and Black Bean Salad

Snack: Cottage Cheese with Pineapple

Dinner: Baked Salmon with Roasted Vegetables

Meal Planning Tips:

Preparation: Plan your meals and snacks ahead of time to avoid last-minute unhealthy choices.

Portion Control: Be mindful of portion amounts to prevent overeating.

Hydration: Stay hydrated by drinking water throughout the day.

Mindful Eating: Eat deliberately and gently, enjoying each meal.

Balanced Meals: Aim for balanced meals with a mix of lean protein, whole grains, healthy fats, and veggies.

Variety: Include a variety of foods to ensure you get a range of nutrients.

Listen to Your Body: Eat when you're hungry and stop when you're satisfied.

Enjoy Treats: It's okay to enjoy occasional treats in moderation.

Feel free to adjust the meal plan based on your preferences and dietary needs. Remember that consistency and a balanced approach are key to managing prediabetes and maintaining overall health.

Conclusion: Embracing Your Journey to Prediabetes Wellness

Congratulations, dear reader, on completing the transformative journey outlined in "Embrace Your Prediabetes Journey: From Diagnosis to Thriving in Health." As you close this chapter, remember that your journey is not just a destination – it's a lifelong commitment to your health and well-being.

From the moment of diagnosis to the final pages of this book, you've explored the multifaceted world of prediabetes management. You've delved into the art of crafting a prediabetes-friendly diet, discovered the power of movement and physical activity, learned the importance of restful sleep and stress management, and embraced the resilience needed for lasting wellness.

Your dedication to embracing your prediabetes journey is commendable. You've absorbed the knowledge, internalized the principles, and taken actionable steps towards your own well-being. Each chapter has been a stepping stone, guiding you towards a life of vitality and balance.

As you move forward, remember that every choice you make matters. Your dietary decisions, your commitment to physical activity, your ability to manage stress – all contribute to the tapestry of your health. By staying informed, practicing self-care, and maintaining a positive mindset, you can continue to thrive and create a future filled with health and happiness.

Your journey doesn't end here; it's merely a transition to the next phase of your life – one where you apply the wisdom you've gained and continue to prioritize your well-being. Be kind to yourself, celebrate your achievements, and always remember that you have the power to shape your health destiny.

We appreciate you joining us on this adventure. May your days be filled with energy, joy, and the satisfaction of knowing that you've embraced your prediabetes journey and are thriving in health.

With heartfelt wishes for your continued well-being,

[Dr.Stephen Campbell]